HOPE MATTERS - Daily Hope Filled Devotionals for Those Suffering from Chronic Lyme Disease and Other Chronic Illnesses

Janice Fairbairn
Copyright Janice Fairbairn 2017
All Rights Reserved
Amazon Create Space Publishing

To my favorite warriors,

Asher and Giya,

who give me hope each day to fight.

TABLE OF CONTENTS

Day 1 - The Journey of Transformation – Climb Your Mountain

Day 2 – Look Up to the Hills

Day 3 – Into Deep Water

Day 4 – Zero Visibility

Day 5 – Overcoming the World While Shackled to Your Bed

Day 6 – Progress or Not?

Day 7 – Hope in Guatemala

Day 8 – Plumber's Crack

Day 9 – Hope in the Middle

Day 10 – He is in Front

Day 11 – God is Greater than Our Ups and Downs

Day 12 – Jet Powered School Bus

Day 13 – The Heart of the Hurt

Day 14 – Old Habits Die Hard

Day 15 – Hope Through the Storm

Day 16 – Making Me Into a Warrior

Day 17 – Nothing Just Happens

Day 18 – What to do with Fear

Day 19 – God is Always There Even When We May Not Know It

Day 20 – From My Womb

Day 21 – Tasmanian Hope

Day 22 – Hope That I Am On the Right Track

Day 23 – Not a Coincidence

Day 24 – Seen Your Tears

Day 25 – Jesus is Enough

Day 26 – Last Call, Stick a Fork in Me, I'm Done

Day 27 – Graduation is Possible

Day 28 – Dark Room

Day 29 – Hope I a Dark Place - I Will Not Be Shaken

Day 30 – A Door of Hope

INTRODUCTION

I am by nature a "wordy" kind of girl and that definitely makes me a nerd to the fullest extent. We toss words around in our culture and they have taken on shallower meanings and it has degraded the purpose of the word. Therefore, in extreme circumstances we have lost the depth of vocabulary necessary to describe complexity to the fullest degree possible.

In chronic illness, there seems to be no modern day words to help describe the journey in its totality and lend weight on the path to healing. One of my new research toys is to use the Webster's 1828 Dictionary to find the original or archaic meanings of words to right the ship in my mind's eye to true meaning of words. Bear with me as we do that with the word HOPE. Follow me on this journey to a new discovery of HOPE.

Webster's 1828 dictionary defines HOPE as the following:

HOPE (n).

1. A desire of some good, accompanied with at least a slight expectation of obtaining it, or a **belief that it is obtainable.** *Hope* differs from wish and desire in this, that it implies some expectation of obtaining the good desired, or the possibility of possessing it. *Hope* therefore **always gives pleasure or joy; whereas wish and desire may produce or be accompanied with pain and anxiety.**

2. Confidence in a future event; the highest degree of well-founded expectation of good; as a *hope* **founded on God's gracious promises**; a scriptural sense.

A well founded scriptural *hope* is, in our religion, the **source of ineffable happiness.**

3. That which gives hope; **he or that which furnishes ground of expectation**, or promises desired good. The *hope* of Israel is the Messiah.

4. An opinion or belief not amounting to certainty, but **grounded on substantial evidence**.

You won't find that kind of definition in today's modern dictionary. We have separated hope from God. The hope of today is more of a wish kind of word, versus the original meaning that is anchored in our heavenly Father.

We are not wishing to get a TV for Christmas kind of hope. It's not desiring a new job kind of hope we are talking about here. We are hoping to get well. To get well and heal while remaining hopeful. Hope is confident. Hope is secure. Hope is well grounded in credible evidence, founded on God's gracious promises. Hope based on this confidence, on this kind of grounding that then produces something. It gives desired goodness, ineffable happiness.

Well, if you are anything like me, then you have never read that word or used it in a sentence – ineffable. What kind of happiness is that anyway? Ineffable means unspeakable joys of heaven that are so happy, they just can't be put into words. (1828 Websters)

From the same source: *Unspeakable; unutterable; that cannot be expressed in words; usually in a good sense.*

This disease is ineffable, but in a bad sense. It's whispered and barely uttered and recognized in our society. It's like a dirty little secret and feels shameful to have. It feels like a cuss word you don't say out loud but under your breath. Like a juicy morsel of gossip that you say out of the corner of your mouth, but never directly out loud.

So, to be grounded in and stand in solid confident hope, then we have happiness that is so great it cannot even be expressed in words. Is that the kind of HOPE you feel? Is that the kind of HOPE you want to possess? Is that the cry of your heart soul to feel immersed in a sea of unending HOPE like this?

Are you with me here? Don't be a skeptic. Don't be a doubter. Take that unbelief and toss it out the window. It is possible.

The biggest dealers of this kind of HOPE are the very people that our culture and our religion would say deserve to not have it at all. Life has dealt them a hand that has been unfair, too hard, too wicked, too much and they "deserve" to be bitter or sad or unable to believe in God anymore. The biggest dealers of deep gut wrenching HOPE are not the fancy pastors on Sunday morning. It does not come from those on the highest of peaks, it comes from the lowly suffering in the valley.

The very valley we would all like to avoid but this life on a broken earth does not allow. These pages of this book are written from these very HOPE experienced valley kind of people. They have bled and suffered and been torn out, thrown down by the storms of this life and depleted until there was nothing but HOPE remaining. But, alas, HOPE remained.

This is the HOPE I want to share with you. A HOPE that is everlasting. A HOPE that shines in the darkness. A HOPE that is confident of goodness coming in a new season. A HOPE that has a reputation and history of success in the highest regard.

There is one more layer to the meaning of the word hope that I must take you through. You see, our English language does not allow for enough interpretation of meaning so we will take it to ancient Hebrew and find another layer.

In the Hebrew, *machaceh*, is used where the translations have put the English word hope. *Machaceh* means a refuge or shelter. God uses the word hope to tell us that within our expectant HOPE in Him, we have shelter, protection and refuge.

*The Lord will be the **hope** of his people. Joel 3:16 NIV.*

*In God is my salvation and my glory: the rock of my strength, and my **refuge**, is in God. Psalm 62:7 NIV*

*I will say of the LORD, He is my **refuge** and my fortress: my God; in him will I trust. Psalm 91:2 NIV*

*Be not a terror unto me: thou art my **hope** in the day of evil. Jer 17:17 NIV*

In Hebrew, there is also another word used for hope. Tiqvah is used frequently in the bible and means "literally the thing that I tie to or bound to, expectant".

*For I know the plans I have for you," declares the LORD, "plans to prosper you and not to harm you, plans to give you **hope** and a future. Jer 29:11 NIV*

*Yes, my soul, find rest in God; my **hope** comes from him. Psalm 62:5 NIV*

*There is surely a future **hope** for you, and your **hope** will not be cut off. Prov 23:18 NIV*

You see, we must be so confident of HOPE that we are literally tied to it as to not float away. It is in the valley, in the darkness, in the suffering that we have the reason to doubt and lose confidence. It is in the valley that we can dismiss the echoes of hope from the past and the faithfulness of God. In the wee small hours of the morning when pain wrenches and the soul longs for death, HOPE is an anchor for the soul. We must bind our hearts to hope so that we do not lose the war.

Read that Jeremiah verse again and read it with hope defined.

For I know the plans I have for you," declares the LORD, "plans to prosper you and not to harm you, plans to give you a tied down, confident and bound to a secure, safe, expectant future founded on God's gracious promises that is the source of ineffable happiness. Jer 29:11 NIV

Wow, talk about a serious promise. It is not hope floating around empty. It is bound to the faithfulness of God. It is bound to the expectant promise of the coming Messiah that came true. It is bound to the prophesy to save his people from bondage in Egypt which he did. Our hope is bound to every single prophesy that has come true in the history of the world written to us in biblical text. And in this verse, he ties that hope to our future days.

Our hope is attached to the truth that came true. Truth that walked. One who claimed, "I am the way the truth and the life, no one comes to the Father except by me."

Let me explain it this way. Hope is part of your stool.

Imagine that your health is a 4 legged stool. Each leg represents an equal platform that your health depends upon to be strong and reliable. Emotional, Spiritual, Physical and Environmental are your four legs. But in a health crisis of any kind, we tend to be focused on the physical healing alone. Physical healing is cost prohibitive, time consuming, exhausting, hard to understand and difficult to achieve. What if we could let the doctors do what they do and we instead focus on healing the other 3 legs of the stool. What if we could impact 75% of our healing for FREE or little cost and those three legs could then strengthen the remaining Physical leg of the stool?

What if on a daily basis, even when you felt physically weak, you could still strengthen yourself emotionally, spiritually, mentally and environmentally? What if HOPE was the basis for that to be accomplished?

What if in strengthening yourself in all these other ways, it eventually helped your physical well being? Like an atrophied muscle, strengthening HOPE takes daily time and stamina to get rigorously strong.

When we have hope we can love.

When we have hope we can forgive.

When we have hope we can laugh.

When we can laugh we can heal.

Brené Brown has found that there is a relationship between joy and gratitude, but with a surprising twist: it's not joy that makes us grateful, but gratitude that makes us joyful.

Hope that brings ineffable happiness. Hope that brings joy. Hope that brings laughter.

Laughter that is good for your health. Laughter relaxes the whole body. Laughter boosts the immune system.

Laughter triggers the release of endorphins, the body's natural feel-good chemicals. Endorphins promote an overall sense of well-being and can even temporarily relieve pain.

Laughter protects the heart.

Do you wake up one day feeling dreadful and burst into to laughter? Nope. Do you wake up feeling on the edge of death and smile with hope? No siree Bob.

Hope spawns fruit that yields laughter. Hope is the seed planted in your heart that grows into steadfast joy, faith, and true happiness. It starts with hope.

When you are handed a life threatening illness, chronic illness, death sentence or critical care issue for yourself or a loved one – the road ahead is treacherous. It matters how you chose to traverse the road. Do you plan on being the victim, mad at the world screaming 'why me?" all the time? Or do you plan on using your faith as a walking stick to lean on and taking one step at a time.

Hope matters. It matters how you view yourself in the illness. Are you alone in a boat with no oars in a terrible storm tossed about by a tempest? Are you cradled in a hammock peacefully below deck in a storm, but gently being rocked and held by the hammock?

Without hope, you are in the tempest each and every time. Without conscious thought, you are being sucked into a vortex of pity parties that will bring all four legs of your stool crashing down.

I cannot guarantee that you can heal by just strengthening emotional, spiritual and environmental situation, but I can promise that you will heal physically slower or not completely at all without the work on the other three legs.

For me, finding Hope each day was a challenge. Trying to keep my eyes focused on Jesus and off my pain and illness felt nearly impossible. It is a journey that takes one step at a time and one moment at a time literally.

This project, this book is a compilation of warriors out there who have made it or are making it day by day hour by hour through the quagmire of chronic illness. Their stories of hope provide a plethora of hope nuggets that you can read for inspiration on your bad days and elevate you even more on the good ones.

It's not how just I conquered the illness and found hope, but how many others, male, female, young and old – all found hope to heal.

Day 1

THE JOURNEY OF TRANSFORMATIONS
CLIMB YOUR MOUNTAIN

"Nothing is a waste of time that adds to the <u>person</u> you are." (Love Comes Softly – Clark)

One of my all-time favorite books is "Hinds Feet on High Places." This beloved tale of a girl and her journey from the Village of Humiliation to the High Places has found its way into my hands hundreds of times. I'm so inspired by the imagery used to describe the journey of the heart that is often an unseen yet important part of life.

Like all of us, the main character of the story encounters testing and trying as she travels in the midst of human weakness, sometimes challenging terrain, and repeated confrontations from long-time enemies trying to deter her pilgrimage. Each time she finds herself at a seeming "impasse" though, something amazing happens – a transforming encounter with the Chief Shepherd. The impossible becomes possible. The disguise of defeat scatters. And step by step, encounter by encounter, this dear girl is utterly transformed from the inside out until she finds herself leaping on the mountains of the High Places.

I was recently thinking about this story while meditating on my healing journey that has involved trying and testing of the body, soul, and spirit on what has, at times, felt like every level conceivably possible. There have been many points where I could see nothing but an impasse…an impossible mountain…a hopeless situation. BUT for the "Chief Shepherd!" One of my most transforming encounters with Him on this journey occurred many months ago as I was facing a particular "mountain" that appeared like the impasse of all impasses. I was feeling overwhelmed and defeated after years of repeatedly doing all I knew to do. The mountain seemed bigger and more impossible than ever and I just wanted it moved!

As I lay in bed wrestling in my heart, a picture flashed across my mind of a breathtakingly beautiful mountain. In the picture I was standing on this mountain where I'd spent years planting grass seed. It had once been deserted but was now covered with lush grass and beaming with life. I immediately felt the Holy Spirit lovingly whisper, *"This mountain is not to be moved but climbed. Climb your mountain, Cherise! In the process, the mountain is transformed, as are you."*

The tears streamed and courage infused my soul. The impossible somehow became possible. The disguise of defeat began to scatter. And something in me came to life as God's transforming power and love enveloped my heart.

Several days later that mountain was appearing like an impasse again. I randomly logged into Facebook and a picture flashed across the screen of when I was rock climbing seven years prior. Immediately I heard in my heart again, *"Climb your mountain, Cherise!"* That picture is now the background on my phone so I see it every day.

I'm still very much on the healing journey and experience those "impasse-mountain" moments. But step by step, encounter by encounter, I keep growing stronger as my Chief Shepherd empowers me to climb the mountain, transforming me from the inside out through His power and love.

"Blessed are those whose strength is in You, whose hearts are set on pilgrimage. As they pass through the valley of Baca (weeping) they make it a place of springs; the autumn rains also cover it with pools. They go from strength to strength, till each appears before God in Zion." (Ps. 84:5-7)

Cherise Krum, Pioneer in Creative Arts Healing, Lyme Disease

https://m.facebook.com/cherise.krum

Day 2

LOOK UP TO THE HILLS

When I finally accepted the disease and looked it in the eye, there was a silent surrender that happened in my soul. That sweet surrender allowed me to hear His voice in a way that I had been missing because of all the fear swimming around me.

Don't get me wrong, the fear was still there and I had to fight it daily, but I could hear Him speak.

On a particularly grueling flight to have CCSVI (chronic cerebrospinal venous insufficiency) assessed, my parents were travelling with me to help since I was in a wheelchair. The flight was awful because of the tremendous cranial pressure I had from the blockages in my venous flow. I was suffering and minute by minute imagining arriving there dead. Then I looked up as I heard my mother speaking to me.

I lift up my eyes to the mountains—where does my help come from? My help comes from the Lord, the Maker of heaven and earth. (Psalm 121:1-2 NIV)

I looked up and out the window to see the foothills of the Rocky Mountains coming into view. My mom was quoting the bible? You have to understand, she had never done this. She doesn't do this. She was a believer sure, but was from a generation that just didn't share faith or words this way. Besides, she also had dementia, so she could barely remember to put shoes on or where she kept the broom. But here she was quoting scripture as a very clear message to me.

The Lord had heard my cries and knew in that moment and on that flight how much I was suffering and He was telling me He was my help. Those were the mountains he created, so He had this covered.

A peace swept over me. The pain and pressure didn't leave, but I did arrive and return in one piece. He had healing in mind. It was a day, a step in the right direction and He was there ahead of me.

Get quiet and listen and allow Him to speak to you. He is there and will never leave you or forsake you. Try reading a Psalm per day and really meditate on the words.

I lift up my eyes to the mountains—where does my help come from? My help comes from the Lord, the Maker of heaven and earth.

He will not let your foot slip— he who watches over you will not slumber; indeed, he who watches over Israel will neither slumber nor sleep.

The Lord watches over you—the Lord is your shade at your right hand; the sun will not harm you by day, nor the moon by night.

The Lord will keep you from all harm—he will watch over your life; the Lord will watch over your coming and going both now and forevermore. (Psalm 121 NIV)

Janice Fairbairn – Author, Marketing Professional, Lyme Warrior and Mommy to two Lyme Warriors

Justlivinglikethiswithlyme.com

$\mathcal{D}ay\ 3$

INTO DEEP WATER

...Put out into deep water and let down your nets for a catch. Luke 5:4

Peter was fatigued, cast down, and fed up after an entire night of backbreaking work. He had been fishing all night and nothing to show for it except for nets to wash, wounds to lick, and aches that only a fisherman would know. Even more, Peter had to deal with all of this in front of Jesus and the crowd that had gathered to listen to Him. Peter was a captive audience in his own boat. He could have focused on his problems, but he chose to focus on Jesus.

Despite all the efforts that Peter put forth by his own strength, Jesus tells Peter that the work isn't over yet. Jesus tells Peter to keep fishing. Peter does as Jesus asked and pushes back out to deep waters, even though Peter knows that fish don't hang out in deep waters at that time of day. What Peter knows doesn't match up with what Jesus is asking him to do. We walk out in faith, and not by sight (2 Corinthians 5:7), and when we do this we act less like ourselves and more like the child of God we are designed to be.

This is a great example of how we feel while we take on chronic illness, stress, and worries. We feel we are on display, nobody could possibly understand our situation, and we have nothing to show for it. Faced with the obstacles and trials, our focus so easily shifts to the problem: pain, fatigue, and debility. We take it upon ourselves to fix the problem and to find the answers. Except, we have Jesus in our boat and He's ready to take us out into deep waters and show us His bounty. Jesus wants us to let go of what we know and what we can see and accept what we cannot see or comprehend. When we choose to remain captive in the presence of Jesus, we are set free from our daily burdens. When we let down the nets of our lives (immeasurable pain, sleepless nights, unexplainable symptoms) we can take up the glory, rest, and restoration that God has set aside for us.

Deep water is where Peter found the big catch. Just like when we get into "deep water", we can also expect to receive the same reward. We just need to trust that Jesus is in the boat with us.

Dr. Aric D. Cox, Hansa Center for Optimum Health, Wichita, KS, Lyme Warrior Doctor

Day 4

ZERO VISIBILITY

Young Florence Chadwick stepped into the waters of the Pacific Ocean off Catalina Island in 1952, to swim to the shore of mainland California. She had already become the first woman to swim across the English Channel both directions. The weather that particular day was foggy and chilly. It was so thick, she could hardly see the boats accompanying her. She swam for 15 hours. When she begged to be taken out of the water along the way, her mother, in a boat alongside her, told her she was close and that she could make it. Eventually, emotional and physical exhaustion set it and she stopped swimming and was pulled out. It was only then did she find out how close she was to the coast. She was less than a ½ mile away.

The next day at a press conference Florence said, "All I could see was the fog....I think if I could have seen the shore, I would have made it."

Call is gloom, smog, haze, murkiness, obscurity, soupy, nebula or miasma and I know what it feels like. Travelling in five minute increments through life because of a chronic health impediment is predictably difficult to navigate. How do you see where you are going, where is the goal, where is the end of it? Where is your lighthouse? What is your compass? How can you know when it will end?

Webster's defines miasma as a dangerous, foreboding deathlike atmosphere. How do you get up to live each day feeling like you are in the vice grip of death itself?

It feels like there is no end in sight. It feels like you cannot make it another day. It feels like you must give up. But what if you are that close, as close as Florence?

I finally figured it out. If I focused on next year or making it to see my kids graduate or to a family reunion next summer I would deflate instantly and want to give up. I had to set my eyes on a simple task in one hour and make it through that one thing. Then I would reset and make it one more hour. Soon, I could make it through the day. Soon I could make it to the next day. That is as far as I could imagine going.

If we are being honest, this battle of chronic illness is more like swimming across the Pacific Ocean. But if we knew it was that far, we wouldn't even begin, let alone keep going. One stroke at a time, one day at a time. We have no idea how far it really is. We have no idea when it will relent. We have no idea when and where the end will arrive. Because of that fact, we must not focus on the end, but the next step. The next task, the next day.

When the fog gets thick and we want to give up, we shift our focus. Shift it completely away from the mundane exhausting tasks of this life and this world and just focus on Jesus. If we are basking in Jesus, then we are less likely to get eaten up by the fog. If we are focused on Jesus then the pity party will stay away. Discouragement is less likely, despair will stay away.

Don't give up, you are closer than you think.

So we fix our eyes not on what is seen, but on what is unseen, since what is seen is temporary, but what is unseen is eternal. (2 Corinthians 4:18 NIV)

Janice Fairbairn – Author, Marketing Professional, Lyme Warrior and Mommy to two Lyme Warriors

Justlivinglikethiswithlyme.com

Day 5

OVERCOMING THE WORLD WHILE SHACKLED TO YOUR BED

"I claim not to have controlled events, but I confess plainly that events have controlled me." -President Lincoln

For everyone who has been born of God overcomes the world. And this is the victory that has overcome the world-our faith. Who is it that overcomes the world except the one who believes. (1 John 5:4-5)

I had heard this scripture during one of the rare Sunday's I was still able to go to church. I had fought against the pain for so many years. But lately I had been unable to lift my arms long enough to wash my hair. I stood their afflicted and weary as the hot water began to make my legs shake even more.

My illness had no name at that time.But it officially had more strength than I did. My body didn't work, and my mind was working less and less. I dwelled on this passage as the water continued to flow. I was too weak to do much of anything, but I did have faith. And this verse says that if I have FAITH, then I have overcome the world. I could no longer overcome the 15 steps that separated the upstairs and the downstairs, but I did have faith. I began to claim out loud that promise.

I then read a book by Charles Capps called The Tongue, A Creative Force. What I began to understand was that our words are the most powerful force in the universe. Our double edged sword. Having grown up in church I had heard people pray for health and restoration all my life. But I had never seen anyone healed in a supernatural way. Where was this BIG God? Where was this God when my water was getting shut off for lack of payment, where was my PROVIDER, my Jehovah-Jireh, the Lord who will see to it (Gen 22)?

As my kids were living with the symptoms of congenital Lyme, where was my HEALER, Jehovah-Rapha the Lord who heals (Ex 15:22-26)? And as I begged once again for mercy from an illness with no name. Where was my VICTORY? Jehovah-Nisei, the Lord is my BANNER (Ex. 17:8-15)?

I soon came across a book that would change the trajectory of my life "You've Already Got It" by Andrew Womack. He too said our WORDS create our REALITY, for better or for worse. As I looked around at my life, regardless of how or why I got here. I knew I could not stay in this reality of illness and lack. Andrew explained that as believers we cry out to God for healing, and yet he cannot give us what we already have. What? Everything that Jesus did for us, was done on the cross thousands of years ago. This statement stunned me. My ongoing prayer was "Heal me, make me whole." Now with this new revelation I could say "I am healed and I am whole."I didn't fully grasped this but for the first time in two decades I had a pathway out of illness. They weren't begging God to provide, they spoke his promises into existence.

 My illness had brought me to a place where I couldn't tolerate the weak principles of religion. I needed a god who could give me VICTORY, and here he was, finally.

Sarah Schlichte Sanchez - Chronic Lyme Disease Survivor, Podcaster, Author, Speaker, Entrepreneur
https://www.facebook.com/sarah.s.sanchez.1

www.LymeVoice.com

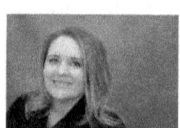

Sarah Schlichte Sanchez contracted Lyme Disease as a teenager, however it took 17 years of pain and suffering before she received an accurate diagnosis. Since receiving treatment at the age of 37, she has devoted her time to help others cope with the daily struggles of living with a chronic illness. She is an author, speaker, and together with her husband Aaron, produces a regular podcast called LymeVoice. They reside in Albuquerque, New Mexico with their five children, two dogs, and 5 chickens!

Day 6

PROGRESS OR NOT?

There are many days that I can listen to the voices in my head and see the symptoms falling down around me and believe there is no progress. Progress used to look different and be defined in my mind's eye in sharp contrast to what it is now.

Progress can mean a moving forward in growth or an increase. So in this battle against chronic illness for three members of my family, I grew dissatisfied and discouraged because many days it felt more like one step forward and two steps back. I grew impatient with progress. I grew embittered that we couldn't make strides for improvement and keep them there. It felt at times like the guy trying to keep all the plates spinning in the air.

Then one day, God spoke to me through his word. I was reading in Philippians and I came across verse 6.

And I am sure of this, that he who began a good work in you will bring it to completion at the day of Jesus Christ. (Phil 1:6 NIV)

I had already been learning that this physical healing journey was as much about emotional and spiritual healing as well as character development in my kids than healing our physical vessels. But as I read that scripture I realized that despite not feeling or seeing progress, God was making progress. He never stops making progress. I can get in His way, but if I am compliant. If I am obedient. If I am willing, then He never stops making progress.

He will bring it to completion. Whether that is this side of heaven or not, none of us will ever know, but from today until then, God makes progress. He never goes into regression. He never backslides. He never has ebb and flow. He never loses. He never has down with the up. He never has one step back. From here until the day of Christ it is all up. It is all progress.

I began to see progress differently. Progress is onward, forward, continuing steadfastly to move. If outwardly my physical body feels no different, I am making progress in my spiritual self. I am gaining in my emotional self. I am believing that my whole self is progressing despite symptoms and feelings. If I link my progress to my faith then it cannot fail, it cannot go backward.

I echo the phrasing of The Message in Philippians 1:6, " *There has never been the slightest doubt in my mind that the God who started this great work in you would keep at it and bring it to a flourishing finish on the very day Christ Jesus appears.*"

There is not a doubt in my mind that God is making progress in me, my kids and each of you. We must get out of His way and allow it.

I have hope that healing is coming and coming in full.

Janice Fairbairn – Author, Marketing Professional, Lyme Warrior and Mommy to two Lyme Warriors

Justlivinglikethiswithlyme.com

Day 7

HOPE IN GUATEMALA

After having a several tubal pregnancies, I had a successful twin pregnancy through invitro fertilization. God told me that I needed to adopt. Of course, we were totally broke from invitro, so we prayed fervently for God to provide and help my husband and I to be in unity about the adoption process. God answered all our prayers and we received finances to adopt our son from Guatemala. I was blessed to go down to Guatemala to live there. My twin daughters and I moved there so I could be a foster mom for our son Mateo until his adoption process was final. What a blessing as I was there to nurse him and care for him so that he did not have to live in foster care or in an orphanage.

Soon after moving there, I began to have some health complications, my face and eyes became swollen. A local doctor had me go on steroids and that did help, but after a few months, I knew that something was terribly wrong. However, I wasn't going to leave until Mateo was legally mine, no matter how bad I felt. Nodules on my arms came up soon before we were to come home. I finally received the results, but they were in Spanish and my doctor was on vacation, so I waited. The adoption became final, my husband flew down to pick up his family!! The day that we signed the papers that I could barely see, my eyes were inflamed and I was losing my eye sight. I already had an appointment for the doctors in the US prior to leaving Guatemala.

I was diagnosed with "sarcoidosis", an autoimmune disease, I had so many symptoms that I went to about 50 doctors' appointments that year. My eyes hurt, my parotid glands on my face were hard and swollen, I ached and was so tired and I was placed on steroids and other harsh drugs to control all the symptoms. Wanting to avoid long term steroids, I began a protocol for pulsed antibiotics, called The Marshall Protocol.

During that time, my faith was really tested. I had brought my son home but I could hardly parent as I was so sick. I had to reach out to others to help me. I continued being on this protocol and then went on to another that was a bit easier for several years.

Despite all the struggles, I just knew there was a reason that God had me go through this. I didn't know why, but I felt so strongly that he wouldn't forsake me and that I was supposed to be mom to Mateo and the girls. I was going to rest on HOPE and believe. I just accepted the journey, but I knew that it would end.

Don't think that meant that I was perfect and that I never doubted. I would allow myself a moment to mourn and be angry, but I would get back up and would move on with faith, I was filled with faith and hope. I never once thought that I was not going to get better. Many times, I wondered why me, but then I think of the goodness of what God is doing long term and how perspective changes and all the people we've had the privilege to touch.

Eleven years after my diagnosis, my daughter was diagnosed with Lyme disease. I did not want her to go down the same path as me, as I had been on antibiotics for 11 years at the time. Every time I weaned off, I would have a flair up of symptoms, the Sarcoidosis had finally gone to my lungs as well. I prayed to God and He answered our prayers by taking her to Hansa Center for Optimal Health in Wichita Kansas. Soon thereafter, I found out that not only my daughter had Lyme, but I did too, likely the root cause of my auto-immune disease as well. And both of my other children had Lyme too. We all went to Hansa and a year and a ha lf later, we are all blessed to be getting better.

I know that there is a reason that God chose this path for me, for us. Most likely it is so we can give back. It has made me a different person, a better person. I am proud of the person God has made me into; still making me into. He is continually working to improve me. I had to let God do that good work in me. I am better today; we are better today and will be better next year. Where would I be without this trial?

I chose to live by faith and not fear. God has used this circumstance and led me to Dr. Caroline Leaf's program (Brain Detox) to help me stay positive and keep all the negative stuff out of my mind. Faith took over through it all, so that the fear didn't win.

For I know the plans I have for you," declares the Lord, "plans to prosper you and not to harm you, plans to give you hope and a future." (Jeremiah 29:11 NIV)

Have I not commanded you? Be strong and courageous. Do not be afraid; do not be discouraged, for the Lord your God will be with you wherever you go." (Joshua 1:9 NIV)

Leesa S. – Lyme Survivor, mother of 3 Lyme Survivors and runs a local Lyme support group.

Day 8
PLUMBER'S CRACK

One terrible day in the midst of the unknown stage of my chronic Lyme illness before diagnosis, I was driving across town to pick up my kids from school. While driving (which is why I quit driving for almost 2 years), I had an "episode". An episode could be described as my eyes going wonky, like a severe migraine and my depth perception disappearing simultaneously. Then my body would get woozy, weak and my heart would have tachycardia and 10 more weird and scary symptoms would occur like my hands and feet going numb, etc.

Needless to say, these episodes freaked me out and I didn't feel safe behind the wheel of a car and with my kids. I stopped at a gas station to get some water and see if it passed. As I was standing at the counter to pay, barely holding myself up, I looked at the guy in line in front of me. He was older, overweight and loud and proud with his plumber crack. He was buying a tube of chewing tobacco, a 40 ouncer and some crappy snacks.

Instantly I'm hit with another attack. This attack, however, was an attack of the "why me". I got self-righteously mad and had myself a pity party right then and there. I had been healthy before the crash. Organic, gluten free, dairy free, dye free – no crappy food – raised our own chickens and eggs – kind of person. I exercised and took care of my body. No alcohol, no smoking, no drugs – period. Why was I the one barely holding on at the filling station and this guy seemed to be doing just fine in his terrible lifestyle?

The relentlessness of this disease could turn me from a faithful warrior to a selfish pitiful baby as fast as you flip a pancake. I would compare my plight to those healthy ungrateful people around me and it would make me so much more miserable.

I am poured out like water, and all my bones are out of joint. My heart has turned to wax; it has melted within me. My mouth is dried up like a potsherd, and my tongue sticks to the roof of my mouth; you lay me in the dust of death. (Psalm 22:14-15)

As I read this Psalm one day, I realized I wasn't the first and I wouldn't be the last. My physical body was so far gone that I struggled to keep my spiritual and emotional self intact. They are tightly connected, as I learned through this journey. I had to focus to keep my emotional self from bitterness, selfishness and rage. You know, really focus, like when you are trying to drive in the fog and you have hands at 10 and 2 and you are almost leaned into the wheel and squinting into the fog.

It was with these words that I found true comfort from the anguish, pain, despair and utter downcast spirit –

You've kept track of my every toss and turn through the sleepless nights, Each tear entered in your ledger, each ache written in your book. (Psalm 56:8 The Message)

Every single toss and turn, every single ache, every tear is accounted for in heaven. Every single one. This was exactly the perspective change I needed. I had to quit looking around and comparing my life to the world. I had to just keep my eyes on Jesus and on his word. He has the comfort you seek. He has the right thing to say. He will put life into better perspective for you to maintain spiritual strength.

Janice Fairbairn – Author, Marketing Professional, Lyme Warrior and Mommy to two Lyme Warriors

Justlivinglikethiswithlyme.com

Day 9

HOPE IN THE MIDDLE

Suffering. Loss. Grief. Trial. Pain that defies expression. These chisel away at us, hollowing out our insides - at times, ripping what may resemble our very selves from us, until it seems that the awful ache is all that remains. A loss far deeper than words can convey. A brokenness that dares not dream of becoming whole.

Along this often agonizing and seemingly unending journey, there are three things God has given me to hang my hope upon.

The first is found in the familiar words of James 1:2-4:

> *Count it all joy, my brothers, when you meet trials of various kinds, for you know that the testing of your faith produces steadfastness. And let steadfastness have its full effect, that you may be perfect and complete, lacking in nothing.*

Did you catch that? These trials, no matter how painful, are the very things that will one day make us whole. As steadfast endurance becomes ours, we are given that which will one day lead us into perfection. Completeness. We will be WHOLE - lacking nothing. Every aching loss restored. All our agony healed. Forever whole. This certainty gives hope and courage as we endure in the present because we know that the very losses and agonies which pierce so deeply now are the very things that will turn and become the seeds of our future restoration and completeness. Our tears are the seeds of our future joy. And we will praise Him with wonder for it all.

The second is that the story isn't finished yet so as hopeless as my circumstances may appear, they do not have the final word. Only Jesus has that. And I can't judge Him based on what I see right now. He's not finished yet. And when He's finished it will be glorious. Or as Louie Giglio has said, "If it's not good, then God is not done." One of my favorite songs reminds me of this precious truth:

And this is going to be a glorious unfolding
Just you wait and see and you will be amazed
We've just got to believe the story is so far from over
So hold on to every promise God has made to us
And watch this glorious unfolding - Steven Curtis Chapman

And finally, I can't tell you just how many times I have felt like the impossible was going to swallow me whole, and I just couldn't possibly make it through what I was facing and experiencing, be it physical, emotional, spiritual, or all of the above. And every single time He brought me through. Again, and again, and again, I found myself facing the dark abyss of despair, and dread, and impossibility, and again, and again, and again He delivered me. I have not yet seen the great deliverance I have been asking for from my chronic condition or in many other heartaches, but I have seen countless, what I like to call "mini-deliverances," where He stepped in with relief, help, and provision right on time, when I thought I couldn't hold on a second longer. If He came for me at the cross, how can He not fail to come for His child who is crying out to Him for help now?

Even as I write these words, my heart is fighting to hold onto this and remember it. And these words shine a beacon of hope to my soul. So, take heart. Whatever you find yourself facing in this moment, no matter how desperate or despairing, He will come for you once again. Look behind you at His faithful track record, never once broken, and stand firm, expecting Him to reach down with mercy and grace right on time.

These are things I hang my hope on even tonight as my symptoms threaten to drown me. These things are making me whole. My story doesn't end here. And He will come for me once again.

The Lord is near to all who call on Him, to all who call on Him in truth. He fulfills the desire of those who fear Him; He also hears their cry and saves them. - Psalm 145:18-19

Charissa Galbraith, Still healing from Post-Lyme, MCS, Toxic Mold Illness, etc.

Twitter: @charisgalbraith

Blogs: https://wordpress.com/pages/treasuresofdarkness.wordpress.com

https://wordpress.com/pages/eilthir.wordpress.com

Day 10
HE IS IN FRONT

One of the ladies in my bible study recently had a dream. She had been struggling with a particular circumstance in her life. In the dream Jesus was in front of her and looking back at her over His right shoulder. She was following Him, but he was clearly leading and in front. He reached back with his right hand to guide her forward following always behind him.

She felt like he was leading her through her trial, her circumstance. She was not walking through it alone. She was not trudging through the trial in prayer alone. She was not beside God in the trial.

He was ahead of her in it. Everything she was enduring he had been there before her and knew what was coming. He was guiding her, leading her, ahead of her.

There is no circumstance of evil or peril in this world that God is having to catch up to or that he can't defeat. We don't have to pray to give God power to overcome. He is all powerful, all mighty, all knowing, the creator of the universe. Then why suffering? Why this disease? Why this evil?

Sin. Sin came into the world and now it is broken. Evil is able to pervade space here but just for a time. Remember there is no time to God and in heaven. He measures time and created time for us to have boundaries. He also did it so that sin and evil would have a boundary. There will be a time of no more sin, no more pain, no more tears. It will end. Just not yet.

Just try picturing it. That each day of this wicked illness, Jesus is before you. He is in your tomorrow. He leads the way. For how much I suffered, for how bad it was, the thought occurred to me that if He was in front, that He could be guiding me to healing, to help, to hope and shielding me from more. Could it have been worse? Some days it sure didn't feel like it could have been, but I know it could. What if it was He that delivered me through the trial, not because I begged Him to, but because He loves me and goes before me to make a path.

What if today instead of praying for healing, you just thank God that He was in this day of suffering before you got here and that He is able and powerful and will lead you to healing. Thank Him in advance for what He is doing and what He will do.

What, then, shall we say in response to these things? If God is for us, who can be against us? (Romans 8:31NIV)

Janice Fairbairn – Author, Marketing Professional, Lyme Warrior and Mommy to two Lyme Warriors

Justlivinglikethiswithlyme.com

Day 11

GOD IS GREATER THAN THE UPS AND DOWNS

A 20-pound bag of frozen chicken in the dryer (it WAS frozen). A gallon of milk in the pantry. Can't remember, did I just go through the bank drive-thru? Brain fog. A new but very real concept had taken over my brain.

I ache terribly; my foot hurts. God please grant me a close parking spot. I hear a knock on the car door awaking me from an exhausted sleep while waiting in the school pick up line. Making it through day-by-day was becoming more challenging. A blood test confirmed the diagnosis of Lyme disease.

My 13-year-old daughter finishes her 7th grade basketball season, goes to bed and misses the next two and a half years of school. Darkened bedroom, unable to walk, sick. My beautiful daughter missing the milestones of Jr. High and High School.

My son finishes his fall tennis season junior year and crashes. I go into his bedroom each morning for nine weeks praying he feels well enough to get out of bed. Is this really happening? Mold nightmares are other people's stories, right? Spore counts off the charts. Thanksgiving weekend we move out for three months as our house is picked apart and put back together. Our whole life was in upheaval.

My stress level skyrocketed. I felt lonely, isolated, desperate, and cursed! That's how it felt. Cursed! Chronic illness, AKA Satan, had a grip. He is a master at intimidation and tried to render us paralyzed as we focused on our health, our mold, our fear.

One day I felt God's tug to do a fast...a 21 day fast. As I prayed and listened, God lead me to the Daniel fast. Through the fast he taught me two life changing lessons. <u>He provides</u>. I knew this. But God used the fast to take me from knowledge to reliance. <u>The second lesson was to consecrate each day to Him</u>. One day at a time. To focus on Him, not the challenges. We were not cursed. God wanted to give me a gift. The gift of reliance. I thanked Him for each trial specifically: Lyme, mold, the daily ups and downs of chronic illness. He revealed He wanted to be more than my God; He wanted me to comprehend He is my *loving* Father. Mine.

The Holy Spirit took hold of me *as I let Him*. He had been patiently waiting. It is true; perfect love does cast out fear. To LOVE God with all my heart, soul and mind allows SURRENDER which results in RELIANCE and from that comes HOPE.

God IS greater than the ups and downs.

Do you not know? Have you not heard? The Lord is the everlasting God, the Creator of the ends of the earth. He will not grow tired or weary, and his understanding no one can fathom. He gives strength to the weary and increases the power of the weak. Even youths grow tired and weary, and young men stumble and fall; but those who hope in the Lord will renew their strength. They will soar on wings like eagles; they will run and not grow weary, they will walk and not be faint. (Isaiah 40:28-31)

Nancy B, Lyme warrior mother of 2 Lyme warriors

Day 12

JET POWERED SCHOOL BUS

There are some things you just don't think will ever happen to you. There are just some things in life you just have to blink twice to believe you saw it with your own eyes.

At a local air show a few years ago I felt this way indeed. The headliner of the show that came after the aerial acrobatics and stunt planes was a Jet Powered School Bus. Yes, that is correct. To all the hillbillies and rednecks in the world, some guy had enough time and money to think, "hey, I should put a jet engine in a school bus and see how fast it can go."

Yep he did. That jet engine was so hot and so fast and so loud, we could feel the heat from the blast as it "took off" down the runway from over ½ mile away.

I thought parenting was going to be different than the life I'm living. I thought that marriage would be different than the one I have. I thought my career would be different than the life I have. Instead of PTA and Martha Stewart, I'm knee deep in a Lyme PhD. Instead of a house paid off and anniversary trips, we bit each other's heads off and are swimming in debt. Instead of a blossoming career, I'm doing whatever jobs I can put my hands on that allow me to still make all the doctor appts and stay in my jammy pants whenever I can't get out of bed.

Its not the life I wanted. Its not the life I chose. It's the life I was handed. I can chose to embrace it or resist it. Hope comes from the understanding that there are things bigger than my plans. There are things bigger and better than the dreams and wishes of my normal heart yearnings. When things were at their worst, God gave me this scripture.

I remain confident of this: I will see the goodness of the Lord in the land of the living. Wait for the Lord; be strong and take heart and wait for the Lord. (Psalm 27:13-14)

So it became my mantra to heal. I would chant to myself. I will be confident that I will see goodness from the Lord in this in the land of the living. So that means before I die. I will and can see God's goodness before and when this thing ends. I can be confident.

Hope is confident. Hope is secure. Hope is anchored to something strong that is only all about goodness. I had to attach myself to the very thought that goodness would come. NO MATTER WHAT. Healing or not, GOODNESS WOULD COME.

So then I had to start looking for it. Amazing thing happens, then you start to actually see and feel goodness happening around you. There is an entire tapestry of goodness that God wove in and around me because of and in spite of chronic illness. It was there all along, I just had to start looking for it.

Janice Fairbairn – Author, Marketing Professional, Lyme Warrior and Mommy to two Lyme Warriors

Justlivinglikethiswithlyme.com

Day 13

THE HEART OF THE HURT

In the midst of chronic illness battles it's hard to see the light at the end of the hour sometimes, let alone the tunnel. But the amazing part is, we have someone who already won the battle for us. It was never ours to begin with. He's already fought and won for us, we only need to be still and trust Him.

That's often hard to do when you're fighting for your life. But when Jesus hung on that cross, He stepped back and trusted His father, OUR father. Despite knowing the pain, despair, and separation that lay ahead, Jesus still chose to obey His Father. I think God even knew it would be heartbreaking to have to see His son torn apart, quite literally, and then have to turn away from Him, for our sake. So we can have a healthy, whole, LIFE-filled life! He loves us that much! He's shared in our pain, He's with us every second, minute, and hour. He is with us every step of the way.

While we might never know or understand the full story in the middle of the journey. I think it's so important to remember how much and how deep His love for us is. He has this victory. It's done. It's over.

Victory is yours, mine, ours. We don't have to fight alone, we don't have to fight at all. His heart shines through in the hurt. It all started back on that cross...He knew about this very moment, when you'd be hurting, and He chose to forget the pain He was going to endure, so He could walk alongside us; and instead revel in the victory He gained for us. He loves you that much. Enough to walk through the fire, to take your sickness, disease, heartbreak, to fully take it, so you don't have to worry about whether or not you'll win.

So you can stand, right now, on His promise, undefeated! So be still today, knowing he's already done the fighting for you, and claim your victory!

His heart is already in the hurt, in the battle He has already won.

Exodus 14:14 "The Lord will fight for you; you need only to be still."

Whitney H. Lyme warrior with brain AVM, recovering alcoholic, singer and composer

$\mathcal{D}ay$ 14

OLD HABITS DIE HARD

I really don't think about it all too much. I've been sober so long, I can hardly remember getting drunk. Sober now for over 15 years, it was a previous life, a foggy memory, a long long time ago.

Then I found myself at a wedding recently. A wedding that had a potato bar as part of the dinner. I had never eaten off the potato bar and found it cute that we were filling our "potato" into a plastic martini glass instead of a plate. The odd part came a few minutes later as we were eating. I kept reaching for that martini glass to take a drink instead of eating my potato out of it. I mean, it was almost an out of body experience how often I reached for it and brought it to my lips without even thinking about it. It had been 15 years. Old habits die hard, isn't that what they say?

These aren't the only kind of old habits that die hard. In this chronic illness I found that my selfishness and ungratefulness would just not stay dead. They were like the bad guy in a horror flick, you could shoot 'em, stab 'em and push them off the roof, but they still came back again to jump out when you least expect it.

Ugh. Every time I thought I was at the bottom of myself, there would come the selfishness to rear its ugly head again and again. Then it would start a cycle of discouragement. The physical agony, the emotional distress, the spiritual separation – it would overwhelm me. I would get in a rut and mumble around feeling and saying, "I will never get better", "I will never heal".

Hope does not get discouraged and does not give up. People. You and me, get weak and we can give up. But hope does not have its origin on earth. Hope is not made in the heart of a flesh and blood man. Hope is heavenly. Hope is eternal. Hope is alive and big and strong and does not fit in a tiny little pocket.

Because you're not yet taking God seriously," said Jesus. "The simple truth is that if you had a mere kernel of faith, a poppy seed, say, you would tell this mountain, 'Move!' and it would move. There is nothing you wouldn't be able to tackle." (Matthew 17:20)

I started taking God at His word. I started believing that somewhere in my body, soul and mind there was a kernel of faith that could be found. I would say out loud "Move mountain".

Jesus replied, "Truly I tell you, if you have faith and do not doubt, not only can you do what was done to the fig tree, but also you can say to this mountain, 'Go, throw yourself into the sea,' and it will be done. (Matthew 21:21)

I would say "Lyme disease, go to the sea." I would yell it over and over while I was in a detox bath. I would speak to the Holy Spirit in me and say "take it out and throw it in the sea."

These were the new habits I created. I didn't know if there was a kernel of faith in me. I didn't feel very hopeful, but I began a new routine nonetheless. I had nothing to lose and everything to gain. I decided to take Him at His word and speak it out.

You don't have to feel strong spiritually to attack the evil around and in you. You don't have to be a mighty warrior of the faith to believe God and have hope to get through this. You only have to have one little tiny kernel to begin.

Janice Fairbairn – Author, Marketing Professional, Lyme Warrior and Mommy to two Lyme Warriors

Justlivinglikethiswithlyme.com

Day 15

HOPE THROUGH THE STORM

While enduring a chronic illness it seems often times impossible to keep a hopeful attitude and to believe that God has a greater plan for all of your suffering. If it wasn't for my faithful prayers and close relationship with God I would have never made it through my dark days. I learned to associate my pain that I was feeling with a greater purpose. I focused my mind on the belief that this pain and suffering is only temporary and it will make me a stronger person because of it.

On days when it was hard to even get out of bed and begin a new day I looked towards God in my time of need and simply whispered to myself "Jesus I Trust in You". Purposely having a positive attitude and finding the little things to be grateful for everyday will lay the path of hope out for you. I realized really quickly that hope doesn't often come in big packages and wrapped in bow, rather hope comes in small doses that add up to be something meaningful and great. Persistent hope in God's plan will lead to a persistent faith life. A Bible verse that accurately sums this up is from Romans 12:12 *"Be joyful in hope, patient in affliction, faithful in prayer"*.

This Bible verse hits on the three essential components that one should have in order to get through any trial in life; joy, patience, faith. All of these are small words that withhold in them a big meaning, a powerful meaning, one that doesn't always seem attainable when we are in the midst of trial. Joy is something you can't go wrong with. Even when your everyday pleasures have been temporarily deprived from you, there is always something that we can be happy and joyful about. It's the little things. Patience is another tough one to attain.

Often times in my life I wonder if God is truly listening to my prayers that I have brought before him. Little did I know, God had a plan for me all along, and He was waiting on His time in order to fulfill my needs. Lastly, there is faith. Never lose faith of receiving a healing from God. Miracles do happen and they often occur to those who kept the faith through times of trial and never gave up. Although you may be in a dark valley now, God promises He will be right beside us to help us through. Faith is finding that light at the end of that valley we find ourselves in, and knowing that no matter what, we are going to make it out alive.

-Miranda Reichenberger, Elementary Teacher, Lyme Disease Survivor

Day 16

MAKING ME INTO A WARRIOR

One day at breakfast, I was reading a devotional with the kids. It had been a particularly tough year for my son. He had bounced back initially after treating the Lyme and other co-infections, but had hit a wall and there were some unbearable symptoms that just wouldn't abate. Over many a night of extreme pain, he had shed tears and questioned why it wasn't getting better. We had prayed, I had researched, we had gone to doctor after doctor and he just had yet to feel relief.

The devotional this day was about waiting on the Lord. After reading the devotional and the verse, I asked both kids if there was anything they were waiting on the Lord for right now. My son quickly responded that he was waiting on healing. Just like you are waiting on healing. You are waiting for the relief to come. You are in that place of believing but doubt has a way of creeping in and questioning if you are doing the right thing, believing the right thing, praying the right thing.

Will it ever happen, will healing actually come?

I asked my son why he thought God was making him wait. Tricky question, especially for a 4th grader right? Wrong. Without hesitation and with gluten free O's bouncing around in his mouth, he answered simply, "because He is making me into a warrior Mommy."

Chirp, chirp were the crickets as my chin hit the ground and tears welled up in my eyes. Silence. His faith just silenced my doubt, silenced my fears, and silenced the crying of my heart to get rid of his pain.

He was wrestling the pain, but he hadn't been wrestling fear or doubt. With certainty he knew that somehow, even though God did not give him this pain or disease, that it was going to be used for good and for His glory.

My mommy heart was warmed and fueled by his faith. The faith of a mustard seed is all it takes and his was the size of a mountain. He wasn't just being made into a warrior, he already was more of a soldier in faith than me some days. His believing His Father hadn't forsaken him and would heal.

In those heartfelt months, the waiting was excruciating, but the healing has come. It has been years now and we remember in faith how we endured, believed, prayed and endured.

No, in all these things we are more than conquerors through him who loved us. Romans 8:37

Janice Fairbairn – Author, Marketing Professional, Lyme Warrior and Mommy to two Lyme Warriors

Justlivinglikethiswithlyme.com

Day 17

NOTHING JUST HAPPENS

During the fall of 2009, my life seemed to be in perfect order. I had just been promoted at work, my finances were in place, my wife and I were celebrating 20 years of wedded bliss, and my 3 children were thriving in academics, sports and their jobs.

The tick borne illness monster crept in my body in a very subtle quiet manner, but within months had taken completely over me both physically and mentally. I went from being a muscular, 175 pound 42 year old man with an athletic build, to a pain ravished, crippled, 136 pound bed ridden man who no longer was able to walk without assistance of a cane and others.

In the beginning, I was bitter with anger at God for putting my family through this trial, and at myself, for whatever it was that I did or did not do to deserve this fate. I felt betrayed by family and friends, as I spent many lonely hours alone trapped inside a body that had betrayed me and kept me imprisoned in a dying corpse overwhelmed with pain. I was bitter at the doctors who were quick to write me off and pass me on to another specialist.

Then one night in my isolation, My Savior crept into my soul, and I surrendered all to Him. As I laid there in agony, crying in the solitude, I begged Him for forgiveness, and for my loss of faith and hope. As I lay before Him, I pledged that all I could give Him was my pain and tears, and that every second in the abyss and every tear that fell, would be my prayer, for someone who was in need of my sacrifice. In the silence He revealed to me my purpose of suffering, and in the silence I felt as a soldier with a mission. I adopted an attitude that no matter what, I was going to win in the end. Either I would die fighting and be with my Lord, or I would overcome the battle with the monster that had imprisoned me and when I regained my freedom, I would offer the key of hope to others.

During this time, I gave up old habits of stressful thinking, bad eating habits, drinking alcohol, diet soft drinks and I took on a daily workout routine and sessions in the infrared sauna. I replaced the daily news with listening to Christian music, and inspirational speakers. I ate, drank, and lived only the pure the powerful and the positive.

During my journey, the 23 Psalm gave me hope and comfort. During the darkest and most painful moments I would repeat to myself, "Yea, though I walk through the valley of the shadow of death; I will fear no evil for thou art with me; Thy rod and thy staff they comfort me."

Then one day my pain and torment peaked, and as the weeks followed, little by little the veil of agonizing pain lifted, and the rest of the year that followed was spent rebuilding what I had lost.

Nothing just happens, for in the spring of 2011 I began to see symptoms in my son, and early diagnosis and treatment meant early recovery. When my daughter became ill in 2012, she too was diagnosed early, and even though it was 3 years before she attained remission, she is living a symptom free life today. Because of this journey, I discovered new faith and a relationship with my Lord I had never known. I discovered unconditional love that was expressed by my loving wife Pam, who took such wonderful care of me and our two children also stricken with this disease. After my recovery, Pam and I started a support group to provide hope and fellowship to others diagnosed with tick borne illnesses, and I have made changes in my life that I truly believe have saved my life and my soul. I have gained so much more than I have lost.

Robert J. R., Police/Sergeant, Lyme survivor, father of a son and daughter Lyme Survivors

Day 18

WHAT TO DO WITH FEAR

Terrors overwhelm me; my dignity is driven away as by the wind, my safety vanishes like a cloud. Job 30:15

My heart is in anguish within me; the terrors of death have fallen on me. Psalm 55:4

Terror, pestilence, plague, dread, calamity, fear.

So, do any of these words describe what you feel within the context of your illness? Lyme disease encapsulates every cell in the body in an all out war. It takes over your emotions, your thinking, your heart, your memories, your mentality and your very soul. It is a stealer, it is a thief. It leaves devastation in its wake at every turn.

So when you talk about it and call it a chronic disease, those words fall flat for me. They just don't cover it. I need a larger more broad and finite word brush to cover and describe what this illness is and does.

In order to better understand scripture and why words were translated as such into our English language, I've begun using the Webster's 1828 Dictionary (online) and certain Greek or Hebrew concordances to find the right meaning of words. I have found it a useful tool to help describe other things about this illness that give it more meat on the bones in conversation and sentences.

Terror according to Webster's 1828 dictionary is described as extreme fear, violent dread, fright, fear that agitates the body and mind.

Pestilence according the same source is referred to as something that produces the plague or other deadly contagious disease. A plague is something that inflicts with frightful mortality, a state of misery, a calamity. Also to be defined as anything troublesome or vexatious; but in this sense, applied to the vexations we suffer from men.

You see, this illness can be a plague that doesn't just want to steal your health, but your mind, your heart, your soul, your finances, your friendships, your marriages, your children and your family.

How can you heal though when you feel this terror reverberating off the walls of your house and your heart? How can you even function, let alone find hope?

You see, I would have never associated the words terror, pestilence or plague with Lyme disease, but look where it came from. I just kept describing it as fear, but then I read Psalm 91 and saw how much description and color the Hebrew language gave these kinds of scenarios.

You will not fear the terror of night, nor the arrow that flies by day, nor the pestilence that stalks in the darkness, nor the plague that destroys at midday. (Psalm 91:5-6 NIV)

The New Living Translation actually says "do not dread the disease that stalks in darkness".

If you continue to read on in Psalm 91, you will begin to feel the Lord taking charge of your fears, your plague, your pestilence and terror. You will begin to feel the momentum shift and boundaries laid. You weren't given a choice on whether Lyme disease would assalt your physical body, but you can decide whether it will take your heart. You cannot decide what friends and family will stand by you and support you, but you can control your reactions to them. You cannot control the brain fog, but you can control your ability to feel emotionally secure in the Lord's faithfulness instead.

No matter how bad the terror was or the brain fog or the neglect or betrayal, I could still praise the Lord, I could still sing, I could still pray for others, I could still love.

If you say, "The Lord is my refuge," and you make the Most High your dwelling, no harm will overtake you, no disaster will come near your tent.

For he will command his angels concerning you to guard you in all your ways; they will lift you up in their hands, so that you will not strike your foot against a stone. You will tread on the lion and the cobra; you will trample the great lion and the serpent.

"Because he loves me," says the Lord, "I will rescue him; I will protect him, for he acknowledges my name. He will call on me, and I will answer him; I will be with him in trouble, I will deliver him and honor him.

With long life I will satisfy him and show him my salvation." (Psalm 91:5-16 NIV)

Janice Fairbairn – Author, Marketing Professional, Lyme Warrior and Mommy to two Lyme Warriors

Justlivinglikethiswithlyme.com

Day 19

GOD IS ALWAYS THERE EVEN WHEN WE MAY NOT KNOW IT

God is teaching me everyday that we have to lay down all of our problems to Him and that He will fight our battles for us. It is extremely hard being in excruciating pain 24/7 but it has allowed me to become closer to God because if God has sent His one and only son on the cross for our sins then I know I can be happy and joyful even in the midst of my trials.

I have suffered for the last 11 years since the age of 17 with an incurable spinal cord disease and was bed ridden for 6 months straight, had 6 epidurals, 7 spinal taps, nerve blocks, 3 back surgeries and now confined to a wheelchair but have persevered and I am now a motivational speaker and my goal is to bring as many people to the Kingdom of Heaven with me.

Through my journey to healing and remaining in hope, God has brought me a beautiful amazing wife and now the birth of our first son. I didn't allow the pain to keep me from life. I didn't allow the suffering to keep me from joy and happiness.

God is faithful beyond what we can imagine.

Have I not commanded you? Be strong and courageous. Do not be afraid; do not be discouraged, for the Lord your God will be with you wherever you go." Joshua 1:9

Allan Schwartz – motivational speaker and survivor

$\mathcal{D}ay\ 20$
FROM MY WOMB

The kids have Lyme. They have everything I have, I gave it to them in the womb.

That moment about 2 months into treatment when that thought occurred to me hit me like a pile of bricks over the head. They had both been mysteriously sick since birth and we had no idea why. The one place I could keep them safe from the world and feed, nourish and let them grow – my womb wasn't a safe place. It was the place I had given them much more than life, I had passed on death to them as well.

The weight of the guilt is sometimes more than I can bear. I wouldn't volunteer again or get in the "give me a chronic mysterious disease" line, but I at least understood. Whether I "deserved" this illness or not, I certainly hadn't lived such a perfect life of servitude to the Lord, so I accepted it. I had not lived clean or pure or without rebellion. I knew some of those choices could have been why I had what I had. I had the faith now and the fortitude to fight and live to see another day, but my kids?

They were innocent of my sin. Innocent of my consequences. They were not mature enough to endure, to walk through this evil wicked disease and all it has to hand out. I would take this disease again and again if I could shield them from ever having any of it.

I know there are more moms, more parents out there who wonder, who wrestle with this guilt. How do you escape it?

I was reading Psalm 139 one day and it hit me. "For you created my inmost being; you knit me together in my mother's womb." God is the creator. He knit them together in my womb. He created them fearfully and wonderfully made despite the environment swimming with pathogens and evil in my womb. They are alive and now thriving because He knit together every cell. He gives life and he takes it away. You see I also miscarried before my first born. I often wonder now, if that child was knit together perfectly for 14 weeks and then God decided he or she wouldn't endure the illness, so the knitting stopped and He swept them straight to heaven.

He knows all and he doesn't make mistakes. He is not subject to the evil and brokenness of this world, we are, but he is not. He didn't allow my kids to be subject to the wicked disease, it was just there in my womb in a broken world. Because he is perfect and able, he knit them together anyway completely unfettered by the pathogens there. He equipped me and has faithfully given me wisdom along the path of discovery and healing. He has never abandoned or forsaken me.

Read it in the Message below until it sinks in and lets the guilt dissipate. You did not do this. It is not your fault. Trust Him to help you lead your kid/s to a place of restoration.

Oh yes, you shaped me first inside, then out;
*   you formed me in my mother's womb.*
I thank you, High God—you're breathtaking!
*   Body and soul, I am marvelously made!*
*   I worship in adoration—what a creation!*
You know me inside and out,
*   you know every bone in my body;*
You know exactly how I was made, bit by bit,
*   how I was sculpted from nothing into something.*
Like an open book, you watched me grow from conception to birth;
*   all the stages of my life were spread out before you,*
The days of my life all prepared
*   before I'd even lived one day. (Psalm 139:13-16 The Message)*

Janice Fairbairn – The Lyme Evangelist, Just Living Like This With Lyme, Lyme survivor, mother of two lyme survivors, author and blogger

www.justlivinglikethiswithlyme.com

Day 21
TASMANIAN HOPE

We had travelled more than half way round the world seeking "hope" and an answer to our prayers for the return of good health for my 24 year old daughter. Wichita, KS was a world away from our country town in Tasmania, Australia, but we felt it was our best chance to save her.

We were to arrive at Hansa to commence our three week treatment. We had everything hanging on this day. Could they make her better? Was it worth travelling so far? Or were we a desperate family clutching at straws throwing good money away and still having a sick child at the end?

We had been battling for 8 years and had come a long way from bedridden teenager to just a homebound exhausted one. We just didn't want her to have to live her life this way.From the moment we walked in the door, I felt it was "right". Whatever it was, I felt instantly safe and at peace. I was feeling calm, but at the same time I was anxious as I needed to know that we had done the right thing.

A woman came up to me and spoke. She was warm, welcoming and had the softest wellspoken voice. We chatted like we had known each other forever. The lady's daughter was also a patient at Hansa. We had an instant connection like no other. I suddenly realized that I wasn't the only mum in the world that felt like this, had experienced this and had felt so hopeless. We both had watched our girls suffer and would have done anything to put an end to it.

This woman, was an angel, sent to protect and guide me when I felt all hope was gone. I knew right then and there that my prayers had been answered. God gave me just want I needed in the comfort and care of a friend. A warm caring friend who restored my hope.

Lindy – mother of a Lyme warrior from Tasmania, Australia

Day 22

HOPE THAT I AM ON THE RIGHT TRACK

I lay in the floor of my kitchen weeping. On my face laid out in anguish and overwhelmed to the point of exhaustion. It was before the ailments had a name. It was before I knew what I was fighting. Both my kids were chronically sick. They were both mysteriously terribly sick. I read, I researched, I bled out both my eyeballs trying to figure out what to do to help them. I am a researcher and fixer by nature and I couldn't do anything to help. I was in deep, scared, helpless and hopeless.

I had prayed for them many times. I had prayed over my kids countless ways. But until that moment on the floor of the kitchen, I had never surrendered them. I just flat out gave them to God. I cried out for wisdom. I needed direction, I needed help, I needed more than I could even put into words.

Did I feel better immediately? No. Did I feel instant relief? Nope. Did I have an amazing Holy Spirit moment? Not a chance. But guess what did happen the next day? God is faithful.

A friend met me for coffee and said, "I felt this morning that you needed to read this book." Really? A book about digestive enzymes. Okay. I read the book and thought – yep I need to do this for the kids. But where was I going to find the time and energy to figure it out? A few days later on a particularly frustrating health and behavior day, I grabbed both kids and marched to the health food store to buy every single kind of digestive enzyme they had in a desperate attempt at doing it my way.

Then I stopped dead in my tracks at the door of the store. There on the door, on a flyer was the author of the book coming that coming Saturday to talk about digestive enzymes and how to get started.

What I learned that day and have used every single day of this health journey since, is that God's way is right and perfect. If I just pray and listen, God will direct my path. He pours out wisdom from heaven abundantly on what to do with my kids every single time since. He is batting 1000. His ways are perfect and beyond our understanding.

"For my thoughts are not your thoughts, neither are your ways my ways, "declares the Lord. "As the heavens are higher than the earth, so are my ways higher than your ways and my thoughts than your thoughts. Isaiah 55:9-10

Janice Fairbairn – Lyme mother of two Lyme children, author, freelance marketing and health advocate

Justlivinglikethiswithlyme.com

$\mathcal{D}ay$ 23
NOT A COINCIDENCE

One random day back in college, I was having a rough time. I can't even remember what was going on or what the struggle really was. Walking to my car I saw a piece of paper just there on the ground by my car door. On it was written this verse from Proverbs 3:5-6 *Trust in the Lord with all your heart and lean not on your own understanding, but in all your ways acknowledge Him and He will make your paths straight.*

It was exactly the message I needed to hear at that moment in my life. It gave me clarity and I released control to Him. This became my life verse; a verse I can cling to, recite and remember who to trust. This verse has carried me through all the troubles of my life ever since.

Even through all of the battle of health and Lyme disease, I would question why this is happening. When I would feel discouraged, I would remember this verse. Trust Him instead of worrying. Acknowledge Him and He will guide me to the right doctor and on the right healing path.

I can research and research, but my ways are not God's ways. It is His path that will lead me to healing and restoration. After my Lyme diagnosis but before I went to Hansa Center, I still had doubts and waning symptoms. I felt I had hit a stalemate. Then I found myself again, doing my own research and I couldn't figure it out.

About that same time, I was getting a new bible and wanted to get an inscription on it. I wanted it to be my life verse, Proverbs 3:5-6. Right before I ordered it, I was reading the verse in my old bible and read past verse 6.

"Do not be wise in your own eyes, Fear God and shun evil. This will be health to your body and nourishment to your bones."

Now my new bible has all these verses on the inscription from verse 5-8. God led me to Hansa center and I am feeling great now. I've turned a corner. It is not my wisdom that has led to healing, but my trust in God's wisdom and path.

This has been a process of learning and allowing my body and spirit to rest and find God's path. I had to let go of my way and my research and completely trust God. He has never let me down.

Trust in the Lord with all your heart and lean not on your own understanding, but in all your ways acknowledge Him and He will make your paths straight. (Proverbs 3:5-6 NIV)

Tammy H., mother, wife and Lyme survivor

Day 24
SEEN YOUR TEARS

There were times I felt like I could literally run out of tears. How was it possible that I couldn't eat food and was dehydrated and atrophied, but had enough hydration to cry buckets every day and night?

'This is what the Lord, the God of your father David, says: I have heard your prayer and seen your tears; I will heal you. (2 kings 20:5)

My husband would say that I needed to keep from crying in front of the kids. I couldn't stop crying for anything. It was just sadness and fear and mourning and pain and exhaustion just pouring from a limitless source.

Nothing gets by God though. He heard my cries for help. He heard my cries for healing. He saw each and every one of my tears. Not only that, but I think he can feel what we feel. I believe, especially for believers indwelt by the Holy Spirit, the Godhead can feel what we feel. I believe with absolute certainty that he knows.

Listen deep in your soul for the voice of God to speak. Listen and watch for ways in which he shows you he is there and is faithful. Someday I should build a timeline of all the amazing big and small things that God did to intervene in my life and health and keep me on the path to healed, whole and functional.

He cares deeply about your pain and your cries for help. He is not idle. He is not ignoring you. He is present. He is able. He is working. He is.

I know it doesn't feel like it at times. I know it feels you are alone. I know it feels like all is lost. Nothing is lost. You are special, amazing and completely loved by God.

Janice Fairbairn – Lyme mother of two Lyme children, author, freelance marketing and health advocate. Justlivinglikethiswithlyme.com

Day 25

JESUS IS ENOUGH

Jesus is enough. Because even if I don't FEEL like it, I KNOW IT!!

Our daughter had tons of issues growing up and challenged our parenting beyond our limits at times. When she finally became physically sick around 16, all the other challenges made sense. She has been sick almost her whole little life. That started the next 5 years of doctors and mysteries and sickness and her just stuck in bed day after day.

Finally we had a name for it – Lyme Disease. But as many of you know, just knowing the name doesn't end the battle. We have sacrificed and spent money and cried and prayed and agonized through this right beside her.

I waited patiently for the Lord; He turned to me and heard my cry. He lifted me out of the slimy pit, out of the mud and mire; He set my feet upon a rock and gave me a firm place to stand. He put a new song in my mouth; a hymn of praise to our God. Many will see and fear the Lord and put their trust in Him. (Psalms 40:1-3)

Watching your child hurt without answers, without the pain relenting, losing her friends, her life has been more than I could bear many times. Here is what I know now. God is faithful. He has been faithful each day, each year and still He is faithful.

"Occasionally, weep deeply over the life you hoped would be. Grieve the losses. Then wash your face. Trust God. And embrace the life you have." John Piper

Being a Christian means......loving, forgiving, loving, showing grace and mercy, loving, not judging, loving.... Being a Christian means being humble, putting others before yourself, striving to be like Jesus. It does NOT mean we are perfect, flawless, holier than thou people. We are only sinners. Saved by grace. Forgiven by our God the Father. I haven't been a perfect mom through my daughter's suffering. But I have always trusted God.

I remember my daughter Caity taking tests from a hospital bed. Today, she is a college graduate. From a Lyme diagnosis, in and out of bed and a wheelchair to working 2 jobs and graduation – we have made it.

Here is what I have learned from this journey. I am stronger than I think. I am not as good a Christian as I think. Attitude is not always enough but a good one is a necessity, but Jesus is enough when I am not.

The bottom line is this. That you KNOW, LOVE, and serve the Lord Jesus Christ, that HE is the very source of the very breath in your lungs. HE is above ALL things, the alpha and omega, beginning and end. HE is the HIGHEST of HIGH, God Himself; and He died as the LOWEST of LOW, on a criminal's cross, so that we can have LIFE and have it to the fullest.

Joni B., RN, mother of Caity a Lyme disease survivor

Day 26

LAST CALL

STICK A FORK IN ME, I'M DONE

In my previous life before marriage, before Jesus, and before Lyme I was a party girl. I spent every night in a bar and every day in a hangover. The term "last call" didn't mean the party is over, it meant "where is the party moving?"

Last call meant a change of scenery, a change of pace or the end of the night. It always came too soon. Always. I reality, it should have come sooner, I should never have been there that long.

In chronic illness, I was always ready for someone to yell "last call" indicating it was finally over. Please someone flash the lights and end this terrible nightmare. I would love to sit here and tell you that my faith never waivered. I would love to tell you that hope never left me. I would love to tell you that I never gave up and begged for death to come. But the reality is that I can't.

I'm as human as you are. This is harder than hard. Tougher than tough and dog-gonned near impossible some days, weeks, months or years. I wept. I pity partied. I complained. I whined. I got sick and tired of being sick and tired.

My tears have been my food day and night, while people say to me all day long, "Where is your God?" (Psalm 42:3)

My bones suffer mortal agony as my foes taunt me, saying to me all day long, "Where is your God?" (Psalm 42:10)

God created emotion. He understands despair, sadness, agony, loss and pain. Pah-lease, our Lord Jesus endured more than we can fathom. He gets it. He also begged it to be taken away, but said "not my will but yours" (Matthew 26) In fact, he was in such agony while praying for it to be taken that he sweat drops of blood.

My soul is overwhelmed with sorrow to the point of death. (Matthew 26:38)

Oh, he gets it for sure. You are not the first one to feel this pull between life and death. You are not the first to want to throw in the towel. You are not the first to yearn and beg and plead for the ending.

Yet, we are not to stay in that emotion. We are to travel through the mourning; travel through the loss, the sadness, the despair. God can help you travel through it and he will meet you on the other side of the fear or sadness or despair and he will bear your burden.

Janice Fairbairn – Lyme mother of two Lyme children, author, freelance marketing and health advocate

Justlivinglikethiswithlyme.com

Day 27

GRADUATION IS POSSIBLE

The past 6 years have been the hardest years of my life. Well, it even goes back before that. I guess I have always been sick or felt bad or been emotional since I can remember. By 16, the sickness had completely overtaken our lives and we had a name – Lyme Disease.

I cannot tell you how many doctors I've seen, how many pills I have taken, how many times I've had needles stuck in me, how many times I've been told I was crazy, how many times I have been in the hospital, how many seizures I have had, how many times I've lost my vision, how many nights I've stayed up crying for the pain, how many nights I considered giving up and ending this nightmare. My parents have spent close to 75k in the past 4 years trying to get me well. We have traveled to Missouri, Kansas, Florida, and California for treatment because the CDC is a joke. Doctors scrutinize you for thinking you have Lyme. People travel far away just to get adequate treatment.

Lyme is an invisible illness. That doesn't mean it's fake. That doesn't mean it's in my head. That doesn't mean I "just need more sleep". It's a very real condition that I will struggle with for the rest of my life. I missed out on a great deal of childhood. I had to drop out of high school and do all my classes and get my GED online.

Despite all this, God has provided a way to heal and a way to live. I would never had believed it if you had told me years ago that I would graduate college. Most days I couldn't get out of bed. This past year, I worked two jobs, graduated college and am pursuing my Master's degree. Who would have ever thought this was possible?

But Jesus looked at them and said, "With man this is impossible, but with God all things are possible." (Matthew 19:26)

This summer I treated my entire family to a trip to Disneyworld. They have all been through hell and back with me and spent and sacrificed more that I could imagine to help me get well. It took two and half years of working and saving, but I did it.

My life has been hard. I've gone through things nobody should ever have to go through. I've looked death in the eye and said "not today". I lost people I never thought I would have to say goodbye to. I've made choices that are not the best, but the one thing I'm proud of myself for is overcoming all of those things.

All I want in life right now is to love myself and accept all my flaws. all my self doubts, my insecurities, my fears; I want to be able to accept that they are there but not let them take over my life and make me feel bad about myself. We can't let our fears define us.

I have a lot I could be afraid of, but I have so much to look forward to now.

As I walked the stage for graduation last month, I'm not gonna lie, I got a little teary. I went through so much hell to get here. I didn't think I would get here. Almost dying 4 years ago to now:.. wow. God is good. All the time and despite the circumstances, He is using it to shape my future and it has made me into the woman I am today.

Caity B., BA Psychology, Lyme warrior, daughter, friend and graduate

Day 28

DARK ROOM

My first job at 14 was working a local photography studio developing pictures in the dark room and other menial office grunt work.

I got my first actual degree in the hard knocks of life working at this studio. They became my family and they sure treated me like the youngest runt. From having me water the fake plants to much more mischief, I got un-gullible really quickly.

Well, not quickly enough. I had been developing prints in the darkroom for a while and then my mentor started training me to develop the film too. For those of you who don't know how this works, developing film has to be in complete darkness. Prints you can develop with a dim yellow light, that after your eyes adjust you can see quite clearly. But to develop film, you can't have any light at all.

As my mentor was training me by showing me a fake roll in the light and then walking me through the steps again in the dark. As he was doing it in the pitch dark, I was peppering him with 14 year old questions. It was then that he told me his secret to doing this in the pitch dark was his x-ray contact lenses.

Now, first of all, the absurdity of that is evident. X-ray contacts would not let you see in the dark. X-ray vision is simply a superhero power to look through walls and such. But naïve little old me, thought maybe somehow without these kinds of lenses, I might never do a very good job at developing film.

Really looking back, I'm not sure how he delivered that line with a straight face and stoic tone.

I feel like tripping through this unknown, unpopular chronic illness is just like developing film in the dark. You can't see a thing in front of your face but you have a task to do. You have to keep researching, keep trying, keep moving forward. There is work to be done. There is no time for training and there are no lights guiding the way. The biggest disappointment of all of course are there are no superman powers to get you through it. No "superhuman ability to survive without sleep" or "superhuman ESP to read the brain and figure out what was wrong".

Nope. So instead, there is something superhuman. God. Hope is alive and well through God. I don't have to have all the answers. I didn't ever know what I was going to do next, I still don't, but God does.

And my God will meet all your needs according to the riches of his glory in Christ Jesus. (Philippians 4:19)

Janice Fairbairn – Lyme mother of two Lyme children, author, freelance marketing and health advocate

Justlivinglikethiswithlyme.com

Day 29

HOPE IN A DARK PLACE

I lift up my eyes to the mountains— where does my help come from? My help comes from the Lord, the Maker of heaven and earth. He will not let your foot slip—he who watches over you will not slumber; (Psalm 121:1-3)

I was dreaming about the song "We Won't Be Shaken" by Building 429 before I woke up, and then this was my Bible reading this morning from Psalm 121. Verse three starts out by saying "He will not let your foot been moved." I love how we can trust Him and His promises even when life makes no sense at all. It echoes the part from the song where they chant "We will trust in You, We will not be moved. We will trust in You, And we won't be shaken"

It has not been only one thing, but multiple, many hardships for myself in this health journey, but also for two of my kids, particularly my son. He is having to start walking down the very path I have just taken and I because I just came from there, I know exactly what he will be going through and I want to take it again for him so he doesn't have to.

I am six months post brain surgery (for an extreme case of chiari). This time last year I felt my life ebbing away, and now, though life will never be the same again, I can feel myself coming alive again! I can feel ME blooming back out from underneath an ash heap! I know I'm still not out of the woods, and may never be, but I'm so grateful to be LIVING AGAIN!!!!!!!!

The hardest thing is being on the line of hope for complete healing or acceptance that complete healing is not a part of God's plan. There have been moments and many of them – still – that I think total healing and restoration might not be part of God's plan for me or our family. Can I, like in the song, Even If by Mercy Me, handle that. What does that do to my faith? Can I truly say what the song lyrics say "I know You're able and I know You can, Save through the fire with Your mighty hand, But even if You don't, My hope is You alone"?

I recently enjoyed painting with my children. Last year today this could have never happened. The road is so long and some days can still feel so hard, as my brain tries to heal, but days like today give me the hope I need to keep on climbing.

> *Grain is crushed, though one certainly does not thresh it forever. The wheel of one's wagon rolls over it, but his horses do not crush it. (Isa 28:28)*

Christ's blessing oft times means sorrow, but even sorrow is not too great a price to pay for the privilege of touching other lives with benediction. We must burn out before we can give out. We cease to bless when we cease to bleed. Poverty, hardship and misfortune have pressed many a life to moral heroism and spiritual greatness. Difficulty challenges energy and perseverance. It calls into activity the strongest qualities of the soul. Like combat, like victory. If for you He has appointed special trials, be assured that in His heart He has kept for you a special place. A soul sorely bruised is a soul elect. (Streams in the Desert June 19)

Tina C. – Lyme Disease, Chiari, mother of 12 and two Lyme and one Chiari warrior son

Day 30

A DOOR OF HOPE

In Joshua 7 you can read about the story of Achor. He disobeyed God and took some plunder from the enemies of Israel and hid it in the ground near his tent. God singled him out and he was killed for his disobedience. It was such a terrible plight and event that the called the place where it happened the Valley of Achor. That name has stuck and was continued to be used as a general term to refer to something troubling, or a trouble spot.

So in response to this story, I'm going to call your chronic illness, your plight, your own Valley of Achor. It is a dreadful plight, forever a smudge on your timeline of life. Ever to be named "illness" or "valley" or "those years I was sick", or however you keep referring to it.

I have a thought for you. Instead of memorializing the bad, focus on the good to come. Read this verse from Hosea and see how God speaks to the people about the Valley of Achor that he knows has now quite a reputation. God speaks to the pain of Achor and the punishment and sin of Israel, but he talks about it in reference to restoration.

There I will give her back her vineyards, and will make the Valley of Achor a door of hope. There she will respond as in the days of her youth, as in the day she came up out of Egypt. (Hosea 2:15)

There is no darkness with light. There is no death without life. There is no sin without forgiveness. There is no pain without hope. There is no punishment without restoration.

For without the bad, the good wouldn't look so good. The good wouldn't contrast and be set apart and be appreciated or noticed. Think about it.

God puts a "door of hope" at the end of the Valley of Achor. A door, an entry, a gate, an entranceway. You can move from the darkness of the illness through the door of hope. The word hope here is the Hebrew "tiqvah" that I mentioned in the introduction. Meaning "tied to an expectation, a longing". Take the cord, hang on and let God lead you out of the darkness through the door of hope.

Janice Fairbairn – Lyme mother of two Lyme children, author, freelance marketing and health advocate

Justlivinglikethiswithlyme.com

CONCLUSION

These stories are real and true and give me such hope. Just knowing these testimonies and people in person has been life changing for me. Being around hope filled people, who deeply understand the layers of suffering and how hard it is to find hope in that darkness. I am blessed to touch and listen to and meet amazing warriors in chronic illness each week who inspire me.

They are the ones who inspired this compilation. My story alone cannot hold a candle to all these testimonies of hope. I am blessed to call them friends, blessed to know their stories and blessed to share them with you.

Surround yourselves with people who have hope. Get rid of toxic people who don't believe and don't see a way out. There is always a way out.

God works His best miracles out of situations that seem devoid of hope…because there is no such thing as hopelessness.

I am so thankful for these amazing people who wrote vulnerably from their hearts and shared the moments that tested their faith and how they got through. Don't be fooled, each of us in this book still fight for hope, sometimes hourly and daily.

We are not all living perfect "as we were before" lives. We are recovered and we are hopeful and we are hope filled. We believe in a better tomorrow. We believe we can win. God is faithful.

Hope lives.

Hope matters.

About the Author

I am a 45 year old married, mother of 2. I discovered I had Lyme disease about 2012, after struggling most of 2011 with severe crashes and health crisis. I apparently had the slow workings of Lyme for over a decade because I gave everything I had to both my kids in the womb. They had been sick since birth and we had no idea what was going on with them. It has been a hard road, one that almost took my life as I hovered under 85 lbs, but it is one that has taught us all great life lessons and strengthened our faith.

As we were climbing out of our Lyme pit in 2013, I realized that God was compelling me to share my journey and give others who suffer a **MEASURE OF HOPE**.

From my previous life, I am a marketing and communications executive and have been a work-from-home and stay-at-home mom. I have now become a PhD in health, healing, living right and all things Lyme. My passion is to see people embrace God's love and faithfulness by providing HOPE for their journey to healing. I love talking about health and healing to anyone who will listen. I adore my kids and how God has used our hardships to grow them into amazing young people with character and perseverance.

softcover book - http://www.amazon.com/author/janicefairbairn

Facebook - https://www.facebook.com/justlivinglikethiswithLYME

Blog - http://justlivinglikethiswithlyme.com/my-blog/

Twitter - https://twitter.com/lymeevangelist

Pintrest - http://www.pinterest.com/jpfairbairn/just-living-like-this-with-lyme/

YouTube-
https://www.youtube.com/channel/UCul1VGlVLd6L0IjDwyPCOXg

ConnectPal - https://www.connectpal.com/janicefairbairn

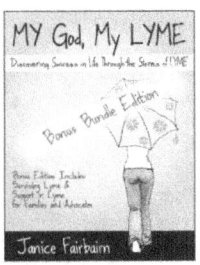

My God, My LYME

Discovering Success in Life Through the Storms of LYME - Bonus Bundle

Also sold separately or as an ebook.

Prepare for a Radical Battlefield. Includes Support in Lyme for Families and Advocates and Surviving Lyme.

Be inspired and encouraged by a true journey of faith through LYME. It's an amazing and real life success story. You can't help but be uplifted and gain strength from reading the story of one mom's compelling journey from the brink of death to healing and restoration for herself and her children from LYME.

Giving people the resources and HOPE they need for healing and how to live until they get there. Whether chronically ill with Lyme, already on your path to healing, or if you have conquered the mountain – this is for you.

Discovering Success in Life out of the Storms of LYME.

Be Inspired and Encouraged by this Journey of Faith

Envision and Experience Whole Body Healing

Prepare for a Radical Battlefield

Get the Emotional and Spiritual Awakening You Desperately Need

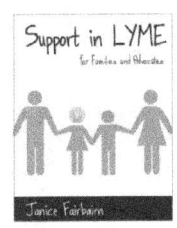

Support in LYME

For Families and Advocates

Also sold separately or as an ebook.

The LYME Diagnosis is devastating for many people who love a Lymie.

What you need to know to survive a loved one's trial with LYME. How to be a parent of a Lymie, how to be married to a Lymie, or how to be a friend and advocate to one. I cover all the bases on how to live through this with someone fighting to heal and live.

What to do when you find out your spouse has Lyme

How to cope with despair and discouragement along the way

Learn how to be an advocate, fighting for your loved one to succeed

Glean support and encouragement about how to be the parent of a Lyme child

Surviving LYME

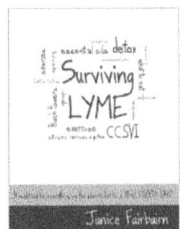

It might not be everything on the planet,
but it's a REALLY GOOD START.

Also sold separately or as an ebook.

Compact and informative without being overwhelming

Changing lifestyle choices in small chunks

Must needs and haves for surviving LYME long term

Do you want to win the battle or the WAR?

The top survival techniques we used at our house to live through the healing of LYME. Using natural biological methods as a framework, these helpful tips have become part of our family's healing and proactive stance against the Lyme monster.

How Many Different Ways to Heal? Let Me Count Thy Ways.......

Over the dozens of Lymies I've met through the past few years, there are common themed questions and areas that come up the most. I've done my best to document various methods of healing, helping, and surviving LYME disease.

A compilation of different methods used to heal, survive and treat Lyme disease based on our family's experience using non-traditional methods of biological medicine.

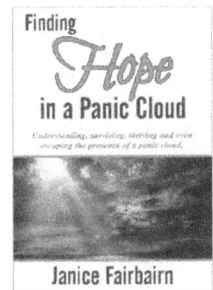

Finding
Hope
in a Panic Cloud

Understanding, surviving, thriving and even
escaping the presence of a panic cloud.

Janice Fairbairn

Finding HOPE in a Panic Cloud

Understanding, surviving, thriving and even
escaping the presence of a panic cloud.

Also sold separately or as an ebook.

- Is the Panic Cloud preventing you from living your life?

- Do you feel that if you have faith you shouldn't feel scared or afraid?

- Do you feel like if you have God in your life you should never panic?

- Do you feel like your faith should keep you from having anxiety attacks in overwhelming situations?

I used to think that I was failing somehow in my faith or that it wasn't strong enough because I felt panic within life's circumstances that were beyond my control. I felt as if I could not breathe at times and that I was destined to live miserable and afraid in a giant Panic Cloud. Sometimes the weights of our trials are a Panic Cloud that envelop and follow you around chocking your faith and ability to live. You don't have to feel that way anymore.

There is hope.